The Good Diet to Ameliorate Your Renal Function

50 Necessary Recipes to Improve Kidney's Activity and Clean the Blood

By

Tiara Crocker

© Copyright 2021 by Tiara Crocker. All rights reserved.

This document is geared towards providing exact and reliable information in regards to the topic and issue covered. The publication is sold with the idea that the publisher is not required to render accounting, officially permitted, or otherwise, qualified services. If advice is necessary, legal or professional, a practiced individual in the profession should be ordered.

From a Declaration of Principles, which was accepted and approved equally by a Committee of the American Bar Association and a Committee of Publishers and Associations.

In no way is it legal to reproduce, duplicate, or transmit any part of this document in either electronic means or in printed format. Recording of this publication is strictly prohibited, and any storage of this document is not allowed unless with written permission from the publisher. All rights reserved.

The information provided herein is stated to be truthful and consistent, in that any liability, in terms of inattention or otherwise, by any usage or abuse of any policies, processes, or directions contained within is the solitary and utter responsibility of the recipient reader. Under no circumstances will any legal responsibility or blame be held against the publisher for any reparation, damages, or monetary loss due to the information herein, either directly or indirectly.

Respective authors own all copyrights not held by the publisher.

The information herein is offered for informational purposes solely and is universal as such. The presentation of the information is without a contract or any type of guarantee assurance.

The trademarks that are used are without any consent, and the publication of the trademark is without permission or backing by the trademark owner. All trademarks and brands within this book are for clarifying purposes only and are owned by the owners themselves, not affiliated with this document.

Table of Contents

Introduction **10**

Chapter 1: Breakfast **11**

   1. Loaded Veggie Eggs 12

   2. Summer Harvest Cupcakes 14

   3. Spanish Tortilla/Omelet 16

Chapter 2: Smoothies and Drinks **20**

   4. Coco Coffee Frappe 21

   5. Rose Hibiscus Limeade 22

   6. Iced Tea with Orange and Mint 24

Chapter 3: Snacks and Sides **26**

   7. Homemade Herbed Biscuits 27

8. Low-Sodium Herbed Grilled Corn 28

9. Creamy Cucumber Spread 30

10. Cucumber Dill Salsa 32

11. Garden Veggie Dip 33

12. Tropical Slaw 36

13. Tex-Mex Deviled Eggs 37

Chapter 4: Soups 40

14. Cool Cucumber Soup 41

15. Pear and Parsnip Soup 42

Chapter 5: Salads and Dressings 46

16. Crunchy Couscous Salad 47

17. Fruited Curry Chicken Salad 49

18. Turkey Waldorf Salad 51

19. Easy Dijon Salad Dressing 52

20. Honey Chive Dressing 53

21. Honey-Ginger Dressing 54

22. Judy's Favorite Raspberry Vinaigrette 55

23. Lime Caribbean Dressing 57

Chapter 6: Fish and Seafood 59

24. Salmon and Summer Squash with Dill Vinaigrette 60

25. Salmon Steaks with Herb Dressing 62

26. Salmon Patties with Pear Salsa 64

27. Mediterranean Style Mussels 68

Chapter 7: Poultry and Meat 70

28. Knock-Your-Socks-Off Chicken Broccoli Stromboli 71

29. Low-Sodium Turkey Burger Sliders 73

30. Black-Eyed Peas for New Years - Renal Diet Friendly Recipe 75

31. Chili Con Carne 77

32. Oriental Chicken Stir-Fry with Coleslaw Pancakes 79

33. Speedy Chicken Stir-Fry 82

34. Spicy Basil Beef Stir-Fry 85

35. Bob's Oven-Baked Pork Ribs............... 87

36. Honey Mustard Grilled Chicken 90

37. Stuffed Cucumber Rings 91

38. BBQ Chicken Pita Pizza 94

Chapter 8: Vegetarian............................. 96

39. Vegetarian Pizza 97

40. Deviled Green Beans 99

41. Gourmet Green Beans 100

42. Green Beans a La Roast 102

43. Green Beans with Turnips 104

Chapter 9: Desserts 106

44. Red, White, and Blue Pie 107

45. Frozen Fruit Delight 109

46. Quick Fruit Sorbet 110

47. Strawberry Sorbet 111

48. Tropical Ice Cream Sandwiches 112

49. Watermelon Ice Cream 115

50. Late Summer Blackberry Tart 116

Conclusion 120

Introduction

Each person with a renal impairment needs a particular diet depending on the issues he/she is facing. It is important to look for a nutritionist to obtain a guide about which food products consume and which avoid or lower their intake.

All the recipes in this book are very helpful to improve kidney's work. So, you can establish a healthy eating pattern combining the different meals.

Chapter 1: Breakfast

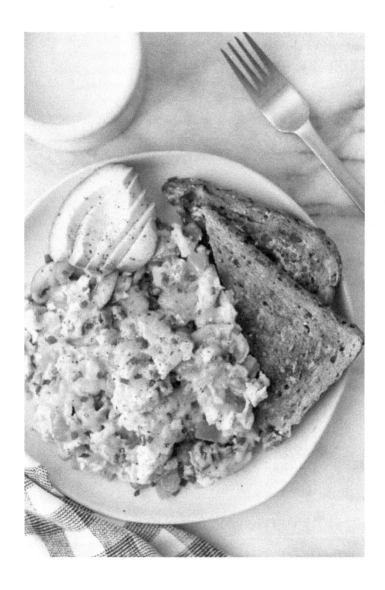

1. Loaded Veggie Eggs

(Ready in about 15 minutes | Serving 2 | Difficulty: Easy)

Per serving: Kcal 240, Fat: 17 g, Net Carbs: 5 g, Protein: 15 g

Ingredients:

- 1 cup cauliflower

- 4 eggs

- 3 cup spinach

- ¼ tsp. black pepper

- 1 minced garlic clove

- ¼ cup chopped bell pepper

- 1 tbsp. avocado or coconut oil

- ¼ cup chopped onion

- Spring onion and parsley to garnish

Instructions:

1. Set aside beaten eggs and pepper once soft and fluffy.
2. Heat the oil in a broad skillet over medium heat.
3. In the skillet, incorporate the onions and peppers and stir fry until the peppers become transparent and brown.
4. Add the garlic, mix rapidly to blend, and apply the cauliflower and spinach immediately.
5. Sauté the vegetables, turn the heat to moderate, then cover them for 5 minutes.
6. Attach the eggs and whisk to blend with the vegetables.
7. Cover it with chopped spring onions or parsley once eggs are fully done.

2. Summer Harvest Cupcakes

(Ready in about 40 minutes | Serving 12 | Difficulty: Medium)

Per serving: Kcal 59, Fat: 4 g, Net Carbs: 1 g, Protein: 4 g

Ingredients:

- 1 tbsp. fresh parsley, basil, and dill
- 1/3 cup diced red pepper
- 1/3 cup diced carrot
- 1/3 cup yellow squash
- 1 tsp. oil
- 8 eggs
- 3 thinly sliced scallions
- 1 tsp. lemon zest

- 2 tsp. mayo

- Brie (optional)

Instructions:

1. In oil, sauté the vegetables until slightly softened. Then set aside.
2. In a cup, mix the eggs and mayo together.
3. Add the spices and green sliced scallions.
4. Add vegetables. For 12 individual tins of muffin, pour in the mixture. Silicon-tins are better on top with a little slice of brie, so the muffins will quickly pop out of them. Alternatively, like that of breakfast casserole, you might prepare this into a 9 by 9 tray.
5. Bake for around 20–25 minutes at 350°F, until each muffin is set in the middle. On

top of each muffin, apply the lemon zest sprinkle.

3. Spanish Tortilla/Omelet

(Ready in about 55 minutes | Serving 8 | Difficulty: Easy)

Per serving: Kcal 265, Fat: 18 g, Net Carbs: 16 g, Protein: 7 g

Ingredients:

- ¼ tsp. salt

- ¼ tsp. black pepper, ground

- 1 large sliced and halved onion

- 1 cup olive oil

- 1 small diced red pepper

- 8 eggs

- 5 small golden potatoes

- Water(1/2 cup)

Instructions:

1. Heat oven at 400°F.
2. Slice the potatoes lengthwise in two. On the chopping board, position the smooth surface of every half and thinly slice them.
3. Cover the potatoes in a medium saucepan with water. Cook potato slices for around 5 minutes, until they are partly tender.
4. Drain the potatoes well and pat them dry before cooking.
5. Heat olive oil over low heat in a medium non-stick skillet that is ovenproof.
6. Add the bell pepper and onions, then stir for 5 minutes. Add potato slices and

proceed to sauté for around 7–8 minutes, until the potatoes are mildly brown.

7. Sprinkle the vegetables with black pepper and stir to blend. Drain out the skillet's extra cooking oil and dump it into a container. Let cool slightly with the vegetables.
8. In a wide mixing cup, whisk in the eggs and salt.
9. Transfer to the pounded eggs with drained and cooked vegetables.
10. Transfer 1 tbsp. of reserved oil to the saucepan and cook over moderate heat.
11. (Keeps eggs from adhering) Rotate the pan to cover the whole base of the skillet.
12. Turn in the ready skillet with the veggie-egg combination. Thus enabling the egg to coagulate slightly, blend for 3–5 minutes with a spatula.

13. Reduce the heat and prepare the omelet for 10 minutes or so. Using the spatula at this time to guarantee that the omelet's sides do not adhere to the skillet. Often every minute or two, turn the skillet softly with the handle to make sure the omelet is free well as the bottom does not stick.
14. While the surface is still a little undercooked, move the pan to the oven. However, you can sense that the bottom is solid. When the top is baked, bake around 7–8 minutes.
15. Remove and switch to a flat plate from the oven.
16. Cover the top and turn it over with one other flat plate, exposing a brown surface.
17. Serve with a salad instantly or reserve to consume later.

Chapter 2: Smoothies and Drinks

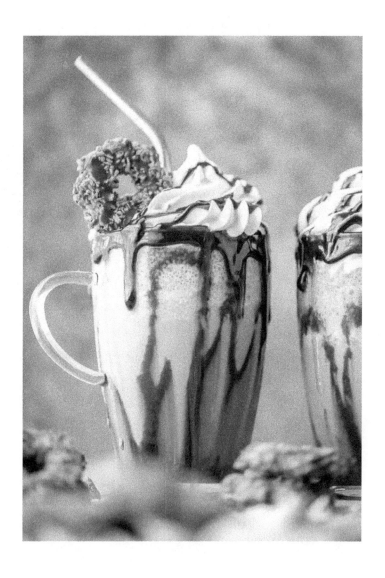

4. Coco Coffee Frappe

(Ready in about 20 minutes | Serving 2 | Difficulty: Easy)

Per serving: Kcal 37, Fat: 1 g, Net Carbs: 6 g, Protein: 0.5 g

Ingredients:

- ½ cup coconut milk

- ¾ cup strong brewed coffee at room temperature

- ¼ tsp. cinnamon

- 2 tsp. maple syrup

- 1 ¼ cup ice

Instructions:

1. Blend all the ingredients till frothy, then pour in two glasses and garnish with cinnamon and serve.

5. Rose Hibiscus Limeade

(Ready in about 25 minutes | Serving 6 | Difficulty: Easy)

Per serving: Kcal 41, Fat: 0 g, Net Carbs: 11 g, Protein: 0 g

Ingredients:

- ¼ cup maple syrup
- 2 juiced limes
- 8 cups water
- 2 pinches freshly grated ginger

- ½ cup dried rose petals

- ⅓ cup dried hibiscus flowers

Instructions:

1. Place water over medium-high heat in a stockpot.
2. When the water is heating, apply maple syrup and ginger.
3. Simmer and reduce the heat for 15 minutes.
4. Combine ginger-infused liquid with the hibiscus flowers and rose petals. Simmer for an extra 5 minutes. To eliminate grated ginger and dried flowers, drain water in a separate pitcher via a sieve.
5. Add the juice from the lime. Serve cold or at room temp.

6. Iced Tea with Orange and Mint

(Ready in about 15 minutes | Serving 8 | Difficulty: Easy)

Per serving: Kcal 18, Fat: 0 g, Net Carbs: 5 g, Protein: 0.5 g

Ingredients:

- 4 tea bags (black)
- ½ gallon boiling water
- 2 large fresh mint sprigs leaves
- 2 large sliced oranges

Instructions:

1. Add tea bags to boiling water and brew till the desired strength. Place in the fridge for about three hours, then add mint and orange slices and let it infuse for some time or overnight. Serve and enjoy.

Chapter 3: Snacks and Sides

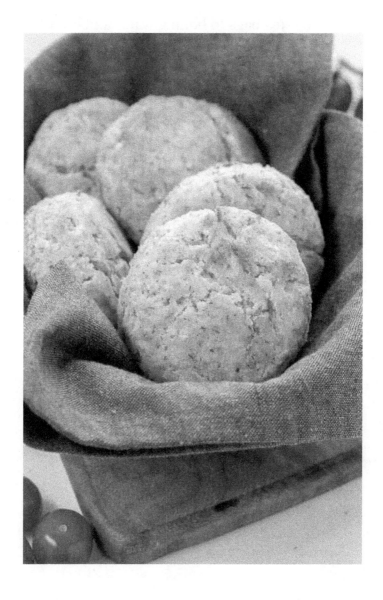

7. Homemade Herbed Biscuits

(Ready in about 15 minutes | Serving 12 | Difficulty: Easy)

Per serving: Kcal 109, Fat: 4 g, Net Carbs: 14 g, Protein: 3 g

Ingredients:

- ¼ cup mayonnaise

- 1 tsp. tartar cream

- 3 tbsp. fresh chives

- 1 ¾ cups flour

- ½ tsp. baking soda

- Cooking spray

- 2/3 cup skim milk

- Rice (1 cup)

Instructions:

1. Preheat the oven to 400°F. Then, brush the cooking spray on the baking sheet.
2. Combine the rice, tartar cream, and baking soda in a large bowl. Then blend with a fork in the mayonnaise, so the paste appears like gritty cornmeal.
3. Combine the milk and herbs in a tiny bowl and apply them to the flour mix. Until mixed, stir.
4. Place on the baking sheet with piling tbsp., for ten min, roast.
5. When available to use, refrigerate.

8. Low-Sodium Herbed Grilled Corn

(Ready in about 15 minutes | Serving 8 | Difficulty: Easy)

Per serving: Kcal 74, Fat: 2 g, Net Carbs: 13 g, Protein: 3 g

Ingredients:

- 1 tsp. thyme dried
- 2 tbsp. minced fresh parsley
- ½ cup unsalted butter
- 2 tbsp. minced fresh chives
- ½ tsp. cayenne pepper
- 8 ears husked sweet corn

Instructions:

1. Batter the first 5 ingredients in a bowl until combined. Spread a mixture of 1 tbsp. over every corn. Individually, cover corn in dense foil.

2. Grill the corn, coated, for 10–15 min over a moderate flame or until soft, rotating periodically. To encourage vapor to escape, open the foil cautiously.

9. Creamy Cucumber Spread

(Ready in about 10 minutes | Serving 16 | Difficulty: Easy)

Per serving: Kcal 54, Fat: 5 g, Net Carbs: 1 g, Protein: 1 g

Ingredients:

- 1 medium-sized cucumber
- 1 tsp. mayonnaise
- 8 oz. cream cheese
- 1/8 tsp. food coloring green

- 1 tsp. onion

- ¼ tsp. salt

Instructions:

1. Set out the cream cheese to melt it.
2. Peel, seed, and finely peel and set aside the cucumber. Mince the onion.
3. In a bowl, combine the cream cheese, salt, onion, mayonnaise, and green edible color, and mix thoroughly.
4. Fold the cucumber into the mixture until it is mixed evenly.

10. Cucumber Dill Salsa

(Ready in about 5 minutes | Serving 6 | Difficulty: Easy)

Per serving: Kcal 34, Fat: 2 g, Net Carbs: 3 g, Protein: 1 g

Ingredients:

- 1 tsp. lemon juice
- ½ cup sour cream reduced-fat
- 1 medium-sized cucumber
- 1 tsp. prepared horseradish
- 1 tbsp. dill weed fresh
- 1 tbsp. red onion
- 1 tsp. honey

Instructions:

1. Peel the cucumber and dice it. Chop weed and onion with dill.
2. Place the finely sliced cucumber in the bowl and add lemon juice to the mixture. Just set aside.
3. In a bowl, combine the onion, dill weeds, horseradish, sour cream, and honey. Combine the cucumber in sour cream mix gently.
4. To serve, store in the fridge until ready.

11. Garden Veggie Dip

(Ready in about 2 minutes | Serving 20 | Difficulty: Easy)

Per serving: Kcal 82, Fat: 6 g, Net Carbs: 4 g, Protein: 2 g

Ingredients:

- ¼ cup radish
- 8 oz. cream cheese
- ¼ cup green onion
- ¼ cup green pepper
- 2 medium-sized cucumbers
- 4 medium-sized carrots
- 3 medium bell peppers (green)
- 7 stalks celery
- ¼ tsp. salt
- 3 medium bell peppers (red)
- ½ tsp. Mrs. Dash® seasoning blend
- 1 cup sour cream

- 1 tbsp. sugar

- ¼ cup cucumber

Instructions:

1. Set out the cream cheese to soften it.
2. Chop the radish, green pepper, green onions, and cucumber finely. The Cucumber Drain.
3. Cut the celery and carrots into strips. Slice the bell peppers into slices with the leftover 2 cucumbers. On the serving tray, arrange the vegetables.
4. Put the sour cream, cream cheese, green onion, radish, green pepper, cucumber, salt, sugar, and Mrs. Dash® in a large bowl. Mix at low speed with blender for around 1 min, until everything is mixed.
5. Spoon it into a bowl for serving.

12. Tropical Slaw

(Ready in about 20 minutes | Serving 6 | Difficulty: Easy)

Per serving: Kcal 107, Fat: 5 g, Net Carbs: 14 g, Protein: 1 g

Ingredients:

- 1 cup shredded white cabbage
- 2 tbsp. sunflower oil
- 1 medium shredded, firm pear
- 1 cup shredded red cabbage
- 1 medium shredded carrot
- 1 juiced lime
- 1 medium peeled and sliced mango
- 1 tsp. rice vinegar

Instructions:

1. In a wide mixing dish, add the white and red cabbage, pears, mango, and carrots together.
2. Put the lime juice, sunflower oil, and vinegar.
3. Blend really well.
4. As a side salad, enjoy.

13. Tex-Mex Deviled Eggs

(Ready in about 25 minutes | Serving 4 | Difficulty: Easy)

Per serving: Kcal 104, Fat: 7 g, Net Carbs: 2 g, Protein: 7 g

Ingredients:

- 3 tbsp. sour cream

- 1 tbsp. coarsely chopped cilantro

- 2 tsp. freshly squeezed lime juice

- 1 tbsp. chile chipotle pepper

- 1 tbsp. minced scallion greens,

- 1 tsp. adobo sauce

- 4 eggs

Instructions:

1. In a moderate saucepan, put the eggs and cover them with water (1 inch just above eggs).
2. Take things to a rolling simmer.
3. Turn the heat off, cover the kettle, and let it stay about 12 minutes. Uh, drain.

4. For 2 minutes, immerse yourself in cold water.
5. Peel the eggs and chop them with a thin knife lengthwise.
6. In a tub, cut the yolks. Set aside whites on a tray split side up.
7. With a fork, mix the yolks in the bowl.
8. Put sour cream, lime juice, chipotle, scallion greens, chili pepper and adobo sauce to taste.
9. When well mixed, mash with a fork.
10. Using a wooden spoon to pound until the yolk mix becomes soft and fluffy.
11. Carefully fill the egg white with yolk mixture.
12. Add new cilantro to the garnish.
13. At room temp, serve.

Chapter 4: Soups

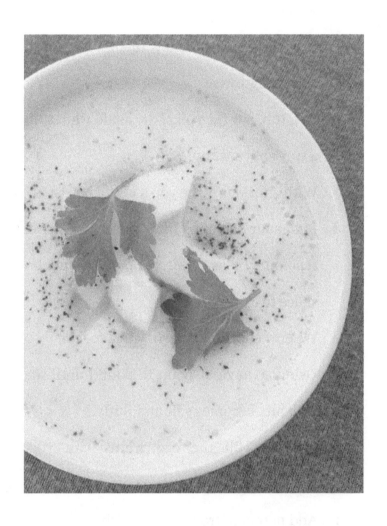

14. Cool Cucumber Soup

(Ready in about 20 minutes | Serving 5 | Difficulty: Easy)

Per serving: Kcal 77, Fat: 5 g, Net Carbs: 5 g, Protein: 2 g

Ingredients:

- 1/3 cup white, sweet onion

- ¼ cup fresh mint

- 2 medium-sized cucumbers

- 1 green onion

- 2 tbsp. fresh dill

- 2 tbsp. lemon juice

- 1/3 cup sour cream

- 2/3 cup water

- ½ cup half-and-half cream

- Fresh dill to garnish

- ½ tsp. black pepper

- ¼ tsp. salt

Instructions:

1. Peel the cucumbers and seed them. Mint and chop the onions. Dill thin.
2. In a blender, put all ingredients and process till creamy.
3. Cover then put it in the fridge until chilly.
4. If needed, garnish the soup with clean dill sprigs.

15. Pear and Parsnip Soup

(Ready in about 1 hour 30 minutes | Serving 4 | Difficulty: Hard)

Per serving: Kcal 244, Fat: 10 g, Net Carbs: 32 g, Protein: 3 g

Ingredients:

- 1/8 tsp. powder black pepper
- 1 tbsp. olive oil
- 2 cups chopped, peeled parsnips
- 1 large peeled and chopped pear
- 2 tbsp. butter, unsalted
- 1 stalk chopped celery
- ¾ tsp. nutmeg powder
- 2 tsp. minced rosemary leaves, divided
- 1 medium thinly sliced leeks
- ½ cup chopped onion

- 3 cups low-sodium vegetable broth

- ½ cup oat milk

- 1 tbsp. honey

- 1 bay leaf

- ¼ tsp. sea salt

- 1 small sliced pear

- 1 tsp. cumin

Instructions:

1. Preheat the oven to 425°F.
2. In a medium dish, put the parsnips. Apply oil, salt (if used), nutmeg, and pepper and cover evenly with parsnips.
3. Roast some parsnips in the hot skillet for twenty minutes. About 10 more mins just

till the parsnips become soft, insert the pears and finish cooking.

4. Melt butter in a wide saucepan over a medium-low flame. Connect the leeks, onions, and celery and simmer for Six minutes.

5. Apply pears, parsnips, bay leaf, honey, veggie broth, and 1 tsp. of rosemary. Cap them and get them to a boil. Bare for 25 minutes and boil.

6. Withdraw the bay leaf. Blend the soup until creamy, in a stand mixer, in clusters, or in an immersion mixer. Apply the milk from the oat and mix for 30 sec.

7. Represent in bowls topped with 2 or 3 slices of pear, dotted with ground cumin, as well as the leftover tsp. of chopped rosemary.

Chapter 5: Salads and Dressings

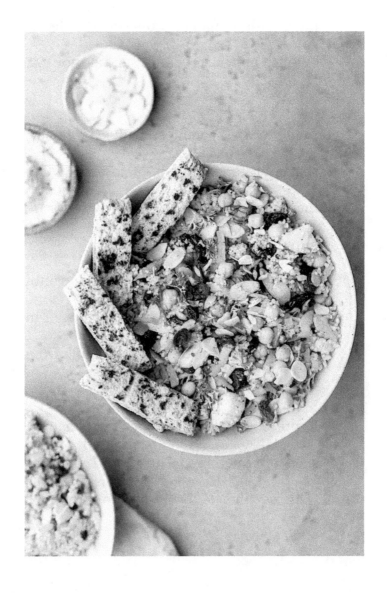

16. Crunchy Couscous Salad

(Ready in about 10 minutes | Serving 6 | Difficulty: Easy)

Per serving: Kcal 121, Fat: 6 g, Net Carbs: 13 g, Protein: 3 g

Ingredients:

- ¼ cup parsley

- ½ cup bell pepper

- ¼ cup sweet onion

- 2 tbsp. crumbled feta cheese

- 1 medium-sized cucumber

- 2 tbsp. black olives

- ½ cup uncooked couscous

- 2 tbsp. olive oil

- ¾ cup water

- 2 tbsp. rice vinegar unseasoned

- ¼ tsp. black pepper

- 1 ½ tsp. dried basil

- ¼ tsp. salt

Instructions:

1. Break thinly and part the cucumbers. Cut the onion, bell pepper, parsley, and olives.
2. Bring water to the boil in a moderate saucepan and add some couscous, back to the boil. Take the pan off the oven, cover it, and then let sit for 5 mins. Fluff using a fork and let the vegetables cool before cooking.
3. To produce couscous, incorporate the bell pepper, cucumber, onion, olives, and parsley.

4. For seasoning, add olive oil, vinegar or wine, feta, basil, pepper, and salt. Pair couscous salad with it.

5. Refrigerate for a period of 1 hour. Serve refrigerated.

17. Fruited Curry Chicken Salad

(Ready in about 10 minutes | Serving 8 | Difficulty: Easy)

Per serving: Kcal 238, Fat: 18 g, Net Carbs: 5 g, Protein: 14 g

Ingredients:

- ½ tsp. curry powder
- ¾ cup mayonnaise
- 1 celery stalk

- 1/8 tsp. black pepper
- ½ cup onion
- 1 medium-sized apple
- ¼ cup red grapes, seedless
- 4 boneless skinless and cooked chicken breasts
- ¼ cup green grapes, seedless
- ½ cup water chestnuts, canned

Instructions:

1. In the salad bowl, add diced chicken and chopped apple, onion, drained chestnut, and celery.
2. Combine these ingredients with the remaining ingredients and toss.
3. Serve right away or chilled.

18. Turkey Waldorf Salad

(Ready in about 10 minutes | Serving 6 | Difficulty: Easy)

Per serving: Kcal 200, Fat: 11 g, Net Carbs: 6 g, Protein: 17 g

Ingredients:

- 3 red apples, medium
- 2 tbsp. apple juice
- 12 oz. unsalted cooked turkey breast
- ½ cup onion
- 1 cup celery
- ¼ cup mayonnaise

Instructions:

1. In a bowl, combine chopped onion and diced apples, chicken, and celery with the rest of the ingredients and combine well. Then chill and enjoy.

19. Easy Dijon Salad Dressing

(Ready in about 3 minutes | Serving 6 | Difficulty: Easy)

Per serving: Kcal 94, Fat: 10 g, Net Carbs: 2 g, Protein: 0 g

Ingredients:

- ¼ cup olive oil
- 1 tsp. Mrs. Dash® herb seasoning
- 1/3 cup rice vinegar unseasoned

- 1 tbsp. brown sugar

- 2 tbsp. Dijon mustard

Instructions:

1. Combine everything together and refrigerate to cool, then serve.

20. Honey Chive Dressing

(Ready in about 2 minutes | Serving 5 | Difficulty: Easy)

Per serving: Kcal 32, Fat: 1 g, Net Carbs: 6 g, Protein: 0 g

Ingredients:

- ½ tsp. sesame oil, dark

- 1 tsp. fresh grated ginger root

- 1 tbsp. honey

- 2 ½ tbsp. lemon juice, fresh

- 1 tbsp. reduced-sodium soy sauce

- 2 tbsp. chopped fresh chives

Instructions:

1. Add all the ingredients together with grated ginger and chopped chives. Use this dressing with salad.

21. Honey-Ginger Dressing

(Ready in about 3 minutes | Serving 6 | Difficulty: Easy)

Per serving: Kcal 105, Fat: 9 g, Net Carbs: 6 g, Protein: 0 g

Ingredients:

- 1 tsp. Dijon mustard

- 2 tbsp. cider vinegar

- 2 tbsp. honey

- ¼ cup EVOO

- 2 tsp. ginger paste

Instructions:

1. In a container with a lid, add everything and shake well. Use with the salad.

22. Judy's Favorite Raspberry Vinaigrette

(Ready in about 5 minutes | Serving 6 | Difficulty: Easy)

Per serving: Kcal 110, Fat: 9 g, Net Carbs: 7 g, Protein: 0 g

Ingredients:

- ¼ cup canola oil
- 2 tbsp. raspberry vinegar
- 2 tbsp. fresh raspberries
- ½ tsp. fresh tarragon
- 2 tsp. sugar
- ¼ tsp. kosher salt
- 2 tbsp. raspberry preserves
- ¼ cup lime juice, fresh

Instructions:

1. In the first seven ingredients, add the raspberries and tarragon. Blend and consume with the salad.

23. Lime Caribbean Dressing

(Ready in about 5 minutes | Serving 5 | Difficulty: Easy)

Per serving: Kcal 75, Fat: 5 g, Net Carbs: 7 g, Protein: 0 g

Ingredients:

- 1/3 cup low-fat mayonnaise
- 3 hot sauce drops
- 2 tbsp. pineapple preserves
- 2 limes

Instructions:

1. Prepare zest from one lime and squeeze juice from both the limes.
2. Add in the pineapple preserves and mayo and mix.
3. Put the zest in it and add the hot sauce.

Chapter 6: Fish and Seafood

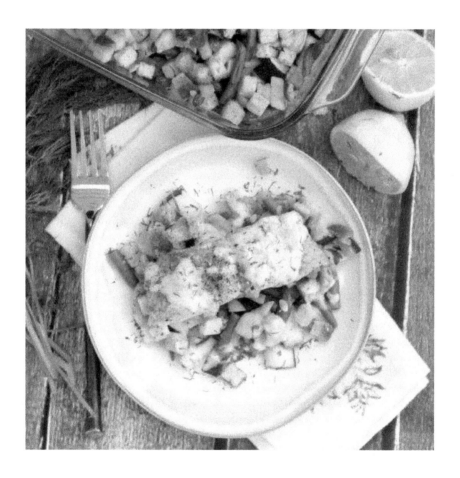

24. Salmon and Summer Squash with Dill Vinaigrette

(Ready in about 15 minutes | Serving 4 | Difficulty: Easy)

Per serving: Kcal 260, Fat: 17 g, Net Carbs: 1 g, Protein: 25 g

Ingredients:

- 2 tbsp. dill weed, fresh
- 2 tbsp. wine vinegar
- 1 tbsp. shallot
- 2 medium-sized crookneck squash
- 3 tbsp. olive oil
- ¼ tsp. salt
- ½ tsp. black pepper

- 1 lb. salmon fillets

Instructions:

1. Shallot chopped and dill weed. Break the squash into ¼ inch x 2–½ inch thin sticks.
2. Combine the vinegar, dill weed, shallot, 2 tbsp. olive oil and ¼ tsp. pepper in the salad dressing container. Just put it back.
3. Rub oil on the salmon fillet and sprinkle with pepper. Using cooking spray to coat the non-stick skillet and heat over low heat. Turn and cook 3–5 mins or till cooked across and opaque; incorporate salmon fillet, cut side down, and cook 3–5 minutes.
4. Heat 1 tbsp. of olive oil in a different skillet over medium to high heat. Add squash, salt, and ¼ of a teaspoon of pepper to the crookneck. For 3–4 minutes, stir-fry until the squash becomes tender-crisp.

5. Strip the salmon fillet from the skin and split the fillet into 4 sections. On a serving tray, place the salmon and squash. Drizzle and mix with vinaigrette.

25. Salmon Steaks with Herb Dressing

(Ready in about 80 minutes | Serving 6 | Difficulty: Hard)

Per serving: Kcal 398, Fat: 30 g, Net Carbs: 3 g, Protein: 28 g

Ingredients:

- 1 tbsp. fresh chives
- 3 tbsp. buttermilk
- ¾ cup mayonnaise

- 10 black peppercorns, whole

- 2 lemons

- 3 tbsp. fresh dill weed, fresh

- 1 medium-sized onion

- 3 parsley sprigs

- 2 lb. salmon steaks

- 2 bay leaves

- ½ tsp. salt

Instructions:

1. Set aside one lemon in 6 wedges. 1/2 tsp. zest of other lemon peel. 5 tbsp. of lemon extract. Cut the onion and chop the parsley and the dill grass.

2. Combine the buttermilk, mayo, 2 tbsp. of dill herb, lemon zest chives, and 1 tbsp. of

lemon juice in a tiny mixing bowl for dressing. Cover and relax for a minimum of one hour.

3. Mix 1–1/2 cups of water in a 12-inch pan, with bay leaves, 4 tbsp. of lemon juice, peppercorns, onion, parsley, and salt remaining. Carry to a boil; incorporate salmon steaks. Encompass; cook 8–12 mins or when measured with a fork, before fish flakes easily.

4. Serve the dressing-topped salmon steaks. Garnish with the leftover dill weed and lemon wedges.

26. Salmon Patties with Pear Salsa

(Ready in about 40 minutes | Serving 5 | Difficulty: Medium)

Per serving: Kcal 290, Fat: 9 g, Net Carbs: 24 g, Protein: 25 g

Ingredients:

For Patty:

- 1 small finely chopped onion

- 2 (7.5oz.) rinsed, drained and canned salmon, drained

- 2 medium lightly beaten eggs

- 1 finely diced celery stalk

- 2 tbsp. fresh chopped parsley

- 2 tsp. Dijon mustard

- 1/8 tsp. black pepper

- 1 pinch sea salt

- 1 ¼ cups homemade breadcrumbs

- 1 lemon, wedged
- 3 tsp. divided olive oil

For Salsa:

- ½ cup diced red onion
- 1 small seeded, peeled and chopped plum tomato
- 1 tbsp. minced fresh ginger
- 1 tsp. mustard powder
- 2 seeded and diced jalapeño peppers
- 2 tbsp. lime juice
- 1 tsp. pepper flakes
- 1 large peeled and chopped Bosc pears

Instructions:

1. In a big tub, mix the packaged salmon, parsley, onion, celery, Dijon mustard egg, and breadcrumbs.
2. Season with pepper and salt and blend until well mixed.
3. Shape the mixture into 5 patties of similar consistency.
4. Heat oil over medium heat in a skillet.
5. Prep patties in groups until they are golden and crispy, around 3–4 minutes on each hand. Drain on towels made of cloth.
6. In a mixing cup, blend together the ginger, pears, onions, tomatoes, lime juice, jalapenos, pepper flakes, and powdered mustard. Stir thoroughly to mix.
7. Scoop salsa onto individual plates with a spoon over or under every salmon patty.
8. With each meal, offer a lemon slice.

27. Mediterranean Style Mussels

(Ready in about 35 minutes | Serving 4 | Difficulty: Easy)

Per serving: Kcal 256, Fat: 10 g, Net Carbs: 9 g, Protein: 21 g

Ingredients:

- 2 tbsp. unsalted butter,
- 12 oz. fresh, clean, raw, and de-bearded mussels
- 1 small thinly chopped onion
- 2 garlic cloves, minced
- 2 cups white wine
- ¼ cup chopped parsley

Instructions:

1. Melt butter over a moderate flame in a broad, deep skillet.
2. Connect the garlic and onion and simmer for five min.
3. Switch the heat to moderate for two min, or before the wine bursts, and introduce the parsley, wine, and mussels.
4. Cover and switch the flame down to boil with a lid. Cook before you open the mussels.
5. In a wide tub, eat mussels within the shells. Over mussels, pour the gravy.

Chapter 7: Poultry and Meat

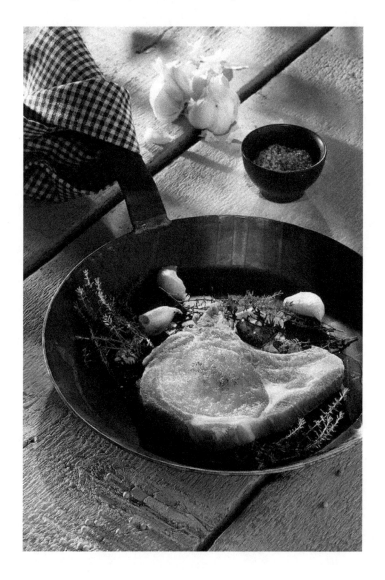

28. Knock-Your-Socks-Off Chicken Broccoli Stromboli

(Ready in about 20 minutes | Serving 4 | Difficulty: Easy)

Per serving: Kcal 522, Fat: 17 g, Net Carbs: 49 g, Protein: 38 g

Ingredients:

- 1 tsp. crushed pepper flakes

- 2 cups chicken breast, cooked and diced

- 1 cup low-salt shredded mozzarella cheese

- 1 tbsp. chopped fresh garlic

- 2 cups blanched broccoli florets, fresh

- 1 lb. pizza dough

- 2 tbsp. olive oil

- 1 tbsp. chopped fresh oregano

- 2 tbsp. flour

Instructions:

1. Preheat the furnace to 400°F.
2. In a big dish, mix the oregano, cheese, chicken, pepper flakes, garlic, and broccoli, and set it aside.
3. Flour dust tabletop and stretch the dough out until you hit a rectangular form of 11 by 14.
4. Place the chicken mix along its longest line, about 2" from the brink of dough.
5. Roll and pinch ends and seam when secured securely (a fork can be used to crimp edges for a tight seal).

6. Using olive oil to clean the surface and make 3 narrow incisions on the surface of the dough.
7. Bake on the lightly greased baking tray sheet for 8–12 minutes on each side.
8. Remove, give 3–5 minutes to settle, then slice and serve.

29. Low-Sodium Turkey Burger Sliders

(Ready in about 6 hours| Serving 8 | Difficulty: Hard)

Per serving: Kcal 85, Fat: 51 g, Net Carbs: 35 g, Protein: 8 g

Ingredients:

- 1 tsp. garlic powder

- ¼ cup chopped white onion

- 1 tsp. basil powder

- ¼ cup chopped green pepper

- 1 tsp. rosemary

- ¼ cup chopped red pepper

- 16 oz. minced turkey

Instructions:

1. Mix the minced turkey, green and red peppers, basil, onions, garlic, and rosemary together in a huge bowl.
2. Shape them into eight tiny patties and put them in the covered bowl. To give flavors time to absorb in the meat, put it in the fridge for five hours.

3. In a wide skillet, prepare the patties over medium flame, rotating just once, upon an interior temperature 180°F.

4. Place them with your favorite buns and eat them when patties are prepared.

30. Black-Eyed Peas for New Years - Renal Diet Friendly Recipe

(Ready in about 60 minutes | Serving 4 | Difficulty: Medium)

Per serving: Kcal 230, Fat: 10 g, Net Carbs: 26 g, Protein: 5 g

Ingredients:

- 12 oz. frozen black-eyed peas

- ¾ cup white onion, chopped

- 2 cup low-sodium chicken stock

- 1 cup water

- ½ tsp. black pepper

- ¼ cup white vinegar

- 2 slices low-sodium pork bacon

Instructions:

1. Cook 5 qt. of bacon. Dutch oven, until crisp, over medium flame. Remove the bacon from the skillet to prepare the onions, keeping the fat and meat juices in the pan. Crumble and put back the bacon.
2. Apply the sliced onions to the cooking liquid in the pan; fry until clear, around 4 minutes. Bringing the liquid to the boil and introduce the water, stock, black pepper, and peas. Reduce heat, then cook for 55

mins or till peas are soft and evaporate with the water. Add vinegar that will lend the peas a gravy-like look. The ladle also comprises of four plate ware. If needed, serve over rice. Cover with bacon that is crumbled.

31. Chili Con Carne

(Ready in about 2 hours 15 minutes | Serving 8 | Difficulty: Hard)

Per serving: Kcal 190, Fat: 10 g, Net Carbs: 4 g, Protein: 20 g

Ingredients:

- 1.5 lb. lean minced beef
- 1 ½ cups water

- 16 oz. blenderized low-sodium canned stewed tomatoes
- ½ cup chopped onions
- 1 tbsp. oil
- 1-2 tbsp. chili powder
- 1 chopped celery stalk
- ½ cup chopped green pepper

Instructions:

1. Heat a broad skillet over moderate heat. Until soft and also not brown, add the oil, celery, onions, and pepper.
2. Add the minced beef and prepare till brown, splitting into tiny chunks.

3. Connect the tomato processor, chili powder, and water. Thoroughly mix; minimize heat to a low degree.
4. For many hours, simmer.

32. Oriental Chicken Stir-Fry with Coleslaw Pancakes

(Ready in about 15 minutes | Serving 4 | Difficulty: Easy)

Per serving: Kcal 183, Fat: 6 g, Net Carbs: 6 g, Protein: 23 g

Ingredients:

- 1 cup asparagus, fresh
- 1 cup mushrooms, fresh
- 1 cup summer squash

- 1 cup green beans
- 1 garlic clove
- 1 tsp. sesame oil
- 1 lb skinless, boneless, chicken breast
- 1 tsp. crushed ginger
- 2 cups coleslaw mix
- 1 tbsp. cornstarch
- ½ tsp. white pepper
- 4 eggs
- 1 tsp. reduced-sodium soy sauce
- ½ cup water

Instructions:

1. Break into 1' bits of squash, asparagus and green beans. Split the mushrooms. Cut the garlic. Cut the chicken into 1' pieces.
2. With sesame oil, mist 12 inches skillet, and cook over moderate flame.
3. Put the coleslaw blend, white pepper, eggs, and soy sauce in a cup.
4. Pour skillet batter. Prepare, approximately 4 minutes, covered till settled and browned. Turn and cook, around 2 minutes uncovered. Keep warm. Keep warm.
5. With cooking oil, spray a big wok and heat on a moderate flame.
6. Stir-fry for around 2 minutes, then add squash, asparagus, and green beans. Put mushrooms and cook for the next 2 min.
7. Apply the meat, ½ of the garlic, ½ of the ginger and ½ of the sesame oil and fry for

around 3 minutes until the chicken is ready.

8. Mix cornstarch, water, remaining garlic, gingerand oil in a small cup. Spill over the stir-fry and simmer until mixture thickens, constantly stirring from 1–2 min.

9. Slice the pancake into 6 wedges and spoon over each wedge with the chicken mixture.

33. Speedy Chicken Stir-Fry

(Ready in about 15 minutes | Serving 6 | Difficulty: Easy)

Per serving: Kcal 279, Fat: 6 g, Net Carbs: 35 g, Protein: 17 g

Ingredients:

- 3 tbsp. honey

- 12 oz. skinless, boneless chicken breast
- 1 ½ tsp. cornstarch
- 3 tbsp. pineapple juice
- 1-1/2 tablespoon reduced-sodium soy sauce
- 3 cups cooked rice hot
- 3 tbsp. vinegar
- 2 tbsp. canola oil
- 3 cups mixed vegetables frozen

Instructions:

1. Chicken rinse; pat off. Break into 1-inch parts of chicken; set aside.
2. Stir the pineapple juice, vinegar, honey, cornstarch, and soy sauce, together to produce the sauce; set aside.

3. In a wok, incorporate canola oil. (As required during cooking, add more oil.) Preheat above the moderate flame.
4. Stir-fry 3 minutes of frozen veggies or until the veggies are crunchy.
5. Take the vegetables out of the skillet.
6. Add the chicken to the heavy saucepan. Stir-fry over 3–4 mins or until there is no more pink chicken. Drive the chicken out of the middle of the wok. Stir in the sauce; add to the skillet core. Cook and mix until bubbly and thickened.
7. Placed the cooked vegetables back in the skillet. To coat, stir both components together. Cook and mix for another 1 minute or until heated.
8. Serve over rice immediately.

34. Spicy Basil Beef Stir-Fry

(Ready in about 1 hour 15 minutes | Serving 6 | Difficulty: Medium)

Per serving: Kcal 352, Fat: 16 g, Net Carbs: 26 g, Protein: 25 g

Ingredients:

- ½ cup fresh basil leaves
- ½ cup diced onion
- 1 ½ minced garlic
- 1 ½ lb. sirloin steak or flank beef
- ¼ cup fresh lime juice
- ¼ tsp. pepper flakes
- 1 tbsp. soy sauce, reduced-sodium
- 1 ½ tbsp. peanut oil

- 1 ½ cup beef broth, low-sodium
- 3 cups rice, cooked
- ½ cup diced bell pepper
- 1 tbsp. cornstarch

Instructions:

1. Cut the beef into parts that are bite-sized.
2. Wash basil leaves, then dry and cut coarsely.
3. Mix the basil, 1/2 tbsp. peanut oil and beef in a bowl if time allows, about One hr or more, cover and chill. If not, mix the beef and basil together.
4. Heat up a wok for 3 minutes over moderate flame. Apply the peanut oil leftover and rub it around the plate.

5. Onion and garlic are applied, mixing several times. Cook for around 5 minutes, until onion, is tender.

6. Turn heat level to a high degree and apply the mixture of beef-basil. Stir easily and apply flakes of red pepper. Cook till the meat is red, around 5 minutes, based on beef pieces size.

7. Stir the beef broth, cornstarch, and lime juice into the soy sauce. Stir in the beef and simmer before it bubbles. Switch off the flame, apply the raw pepper and quickly serve over the rice.

35. Bob's Oven-Baked Pork Ribs

(Ready in about 6 hours 10 minutes | Serving 6 | Difficulty: Hard)

Per serving: Kcal 268, Fat: 16 g, Net Carbs: 7 g, Protein: 23 g

Ingredients:

- 1 red apple, medium
- 1 tbsp. brown sugar
- 3 lb. pork ribs baby back
- 1 tsp. Creole seasoning
- 1/3 cup barbecue sauce, prepared
- 1 ½ tbsp. olive oil
- ½ cup water
- 1 onion, large

Instructions:

1. Preheat the oven at 225°F.

2. Break the onion into slices of 1/2" slices. Core apple, then slice into 1/2".
3. In a shallow cup, combine the brown sugar and the Creole seasoning; set aside.
4. In the 9" x 13" baking dish, put the ribs.
5. Utilizing brown sugar and Creole seasoning, mix to rub olive oil on both sides of the ribs, then repeat.
6. Place slices of apples and onions on top of the ribs.
7. Load ½ cup of water into the dish and firmly cover it with foil.
8. Bake for 6 hours, roughly. Break the foil with 1/3 cup of barbecue sauce and wash the ribs. Cook uncovered at 325°F for an extra 45 minutes or so before rib temperature exceeds 185°F.
9. From the oven. Remove. Drain the liquid slowly, then remove the apples and onions.

10. Break the ribs into individual parts and serve directly for a later date, or cool and freeze.

36. Honey Mustard Grilled Chicken

(Ready in about 25 minutes | Serving 4 | Difficulty: Easy)

Per serving: Kcal 282, Fat: 18 g, Net Carbs: 5 g, Protein: 25 g

Ingredients:

- 1 lb skinless, boneless, chicken breasts
- 1 tsp. cider vinegar
- 1 tbsp. honey
- 2 chopped green onions

- 1 ½ tbsp. mustard deli-style

- 1/3 cup mayonnaise

Instructions:

1. Combine the mayo, honey, mustard, vinegar and green onions in a tiny bowl to produce a sauce. To eat with cooked poultry, save 1/4 cup.
2. Over medium fire, grill 1 lb of skinless, boneless chicken. Brush with the sauce, then flip until the chicken is finished cooking over many times.
3. Remove from the grill and eat with the sauce reserved.

37. Stuffed Cucumber Rings

(Ready in about 20 minutes | Serving 8 | Difficulty: Easy)

Per serving: Kcal 162, Fat: 10 g, Net Carbs: 5 g, Protein: 13 g

Ingredients:

- 1 tbsp. garlic powder
- 1 lb. minced pork
- 1 egg
- 2 tsp. sugar
- 2 cucumbers
- 1 tsp. cornstarch
- 3 tbsp. red wine
- 1 ½ tbsp. Lemon Pepper Mrs. Dash® seasoning blend
- 1 tbsp. minced ginger fresh

- 1 ½ tbsp. Chicken Grilling Mrs. Dash® Blend
- ¼ cup water
- 1 tsp. dried basil
- 1 tsp. dried parsley

Instructions:

1. Peel the cucumbers and horizontally split each cucumber into 4 circular bits. To get it empty in the middle, extract seeds from the center of each circular cucumber.
2. Mix the ground beef with the cornstarch, egg, wine, sugar, garlic powder, Mrs. Dash®, ginger, parsley, and basil in a mixing cup.

3. Gradually apply 1/4 cup water to the mixture of ground meat and blend well before the water has evaporated.
4. Stuff the ground cucumber with a filling of ground meat. Place all pieces in a steamer and steam until the meat is ready, around 15 minutes.

38. BBQ Chicken Pita Pizza

(Ready in about 15 minutes | Serving 2 | Difficulty: Easy)

Per serving: Kcal 320, Fat: 9 g, Net Carbs: 34 g, Protein: 23 g

Ingredients:

- 3 tbsp. barbecue sauce, low-sodium

- 4 oz. cooked chicken

- ¼ cup purple onion

- 1/8 tsp. garlic powder

- 2 tbsp. feta cheese, crumbled

- 2 (6 ½") pita bread

- Non-stick cooking spray

Instructions:

1. Preheat the oven at 350°F.
2. Using non-stick spray to spray the baking sheet and put 2 pitas on the sheet.
3. Cover each pita with 1–1/2 tbsp. of BBQ sauce.
4. Spread the onion and slice over the pitas.
5. Chicken cubes and scatter over pitas.
6. Toss garlic powder and feta cheese over the pitas.
7. Cook for between 11 and 13 minutes.

Chapter 8: Vegetarian

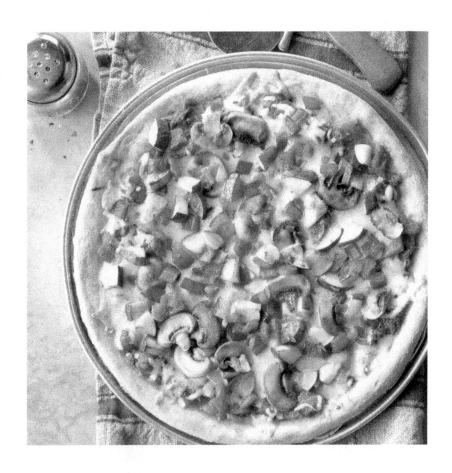

39. Vegetarian Pizza

(Ready in about 25 minutes | Serving 8 | Difficulty: Easy)

Per serving: Kcal 289, Fat: 12 g, Net Carbs: 35 g, Protein: 8 g

Ingredients:

- ½ cup shredded part-skim mozzarella cheese
- ½ cup bell pepper
- ½ cup tidbits pineapple
- Pizza Dough (15 inch)
- ½ cup mushroom
- 2 tbsp. Parmesan cheese grated
- 1 cup red pepper roasted tomato sauce

- ½ cup red onion

Instructions:

1. Chop the bell pepper; slice the onion.
2. Preheat the oven at 425°F.
3. To produce two flat 12" pizza crusts, form the pizza dough.
4. Spread over each pizza with 1/2 cup tomato sauce.
5. Garnish with mushrooms, red onion, pineapple and bell pepper.
6. Sprinkle the top with mozzarella and Parmesan cheese.
7. Bake until bubbly and browned between 12–6 mins.

40. Deviled Green Beans

(Ready in about 10 minutes | Serving 4 | Difficulty: Easy)

Per serving: Kcal 71, Fat: 5 g, Net Carbs: 4 g, Protein: 1 g

Ingredients:

- 1 tsp. Worcestershire sauce
- 5 tsp. unsalted margarine
- 1 tbsp. bread crumbs, seasoned
- 2 tsp. mustard
- ½ tsp. black pepper
- 2 cups green beans, frozen

Instructions:

1. As indicated on the container, cook the green beans.
2. Blend mustard, pepper, 2 tsp. of heated margarine, and Worcestershire sauce together to make a sauce. Warm-up for 30 sec in the microwave.
3. Toss the spicy fried green beans with the sauce.
4. Mix the leftover (melted) margarine with the bread crumbs. Scatter Over the beans, and eat.

41. Gourmet Green Beans

(Ready in about 10 minutes | Serving 4 | Difficulty: Easy)

Per serving: Kcal 67, Fat: 3 g, Net Carbs: 4 g, Protein: 2 g

Ingredients:

- ¼ tsp. black pepper
- 10 oz. green beans, frozen
- 1 tsp. dried parsley
- ½ cup bell pepper
- ¼ cup onion
- 1 tsp. dill weed, dried
- 4 tsp. margarine

Instructions:

1. Cook the green beans until soft in hot water. Drain.
2. Chop the bell pepper and onion.
3. On medium fire, put the skillet, add the margarine, then sauté the bell pepper, onion, dill and parsley once tender.

4. In the skillet, add the green beans and cook until the beans become hot.

5. Toss and serve with some black pepper.

42. Green Beans a La Roast

(Ready in about 25 minutes | Serving 4 | Difficulty: Easy)

Per serving: Kcal 70, Fat: 5 g, Net Carbs: 1 g, Protein: 2 g

Ingredients:

- ¼ tsp. black pepper
- 1 ½ tbsp. olive oil
- 1 lb. green beans fresh

Instructions:

1. Preheat the oven at 450°F.
2. Clean the green beans and finish with the trim.
3. Cover an aluminum foil with a lined baking surface and spread the beans on the foil.
4. Pour over the beans with olive oil and mix gently to cover the beans uniformly.
5. Roast for Ten minutes in the oven.
6. Take the baking tray from the oven and evenly redistribute the beans.
7. Return to the oven and cook for another ten min or till the beans have some golden brown regions.
8. Take from the oven, season, and top with pepper.

43. Green Beans with Turnips

(Ready in about 20 minutes | Serving 8 | Difficulty: Easy)

Per serving: Kcal 58, Fat: 3 g, Net Carbs: 4 g, Protein: 1 g

Ingredients:

- 1 lb. green beans fresh
- 2 turnips medium
- 2 garlic cloves
- 1 tbsp. unsalted butter
- ½ tsp. black pepper
- ¼ tsp. salt
- ¼ tsp. paprika

Instructions:

1. Strip green beans from the edges and break in 1 ½" bits. Remove turnips peel and dice 8 pieces each. Mince the cloves of garlic."
2. Put in a moderate pot with veggies and garlic. Cover and let boil the 3 cups of water. Decrease to moderate flame and simmer for 15 min uncovered.
3. Remove from the heat and extract the water from the container. Add the butter, salt, and pepper. To combine flavorings with veggies, toss gently. Serve wet.
4. Remove and top with paprika to serve.

Chapter 9:

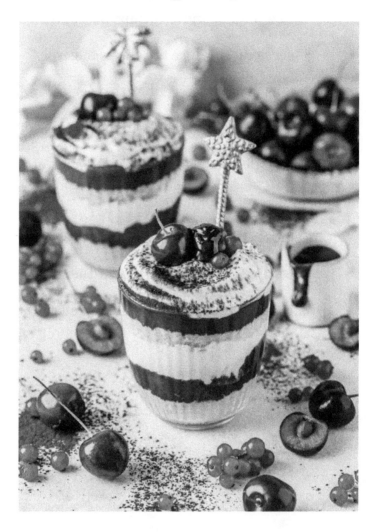

44. Red, White, and Blue Pie

(Ready in about 35 minutes | Serving 8 | Difficulty: Easy)

Per serving: Kcal 237, Fat: 9 g, Net Carbs: 32 g, Protein: 4 g

Ingredients:

- 9" crust graham cracker
- ½ cup red raspberry, low-sugar preserves
- 1 ½ cup raspberries, fresh
- 3 cups dairy Reddi-Wip® whipped topping
- 8 oz. low-fat whipped cream cheese
- 1 cup blueberries, fresh

Instructions:

1. Beat whipped cheese and conserve until fluffy with an immersion blender at medium speed to create the filling.
2. Wrap whipped topping with a combination of cream cheese.
3. Layer the filling uniformly over the cracker crust's rim.
4. Chill in the fridge or freezer for 30 minutes at least.
5. Arrange the blueberries throughout the outer circle of the pie before serving. Layer the raspberries along the pie's inner ring.
6. Complete decorating in the middle with a spoonful of whipped cream and on top with a strawberry or raspberry.

45. Frozen Fruit Delight

(Ready in about 3 hours | Serving 10 | Difficulty: Hard)

Per serving: Kcal 133, Fat: 5 g, Net Carbs: 20 g, Protein: 1 g

Ingredients:

- 1 cup strawberries, sliced
- 8 oz. crushed canned pineapple
- 1 tbsp. lemon juice
- 1/3 cup maraschino cherries
- 8 oz. sour cream, reduced-fat
- 3 cups dairy Reddi-Wip® whipped topping
- ½ cup sugar
- 1/8 tsp. salt

Instructions:

1. Drain the pineapple and chop the cherries.
2. In a moderate cup, put all ingredients, excluding whipped topping, and mix till it's combined. Fold into the whipped topping.
3. Then put the mixture in a tub of plastic, then freeze for 3 hours before it is hardened.

46. Quick Fruit Sorbet

(Ready in about 5 minutes | Serving 8 | Difficulty: Easy)

Per serving: Kcal 71, Fat: 0 g, Net Carbs: 14 g, Protein: 0 g

Ingredients:

- 1 cup unsweetened frozen raspberries

- 4 pitted plums

- 20 oz. frozen crushed pineapple, juice-packed, canned

Instructions:

1. Sufficiently Defrost Pineapple to take out of the can.
2. Put all the fruit in the food processor before pureed and refined.
3. Serve instantly or disperse and freeze in an 8" by 8" container.

47. Strawberry Sorbet

(Ready in about 2 minutes | Serving 4 | Difficulty: Easy)

Per serving: Kcal 22, Fat: 0 g, Net Carbs: 3 g, Protein: 0 g

Ingredients:

- 1 ¼ cup ice
- 1 cup fresh or frozen strawberries
- ¼ cup water
- 1 tbsp. lemon juice

Instructions:

1. Blend all the ingredients in the blender and serve.

48. Tropical Ice Cream Sandwiches

(Ready in about 8 hours | Serving 15 | Difficulty: Hard)

Per serving: Kcal 139, Fat: 1 g, Net Carbs: 17 g, Protein: 10 g

Ingredients:

- 8 packs No Calorie Splenda® Sweetener
- 1 pack unflavored Knox® gelatin
- 1 cup dairy Reddi-Wip® whipped topping
- 15 oz. crushed pineapple canned in juice
- 1 ½ cups protein powder Procel®
- 30 squares graham cracker

Instructions:

1. Cover a 13" by 9 ½" baking pan using a plastic wrap that helps both sides of the pan to hang at least 10".
2. Arrange and set aside fifteen graham cracker pieces in the pan.

3. Drain the pineapple and put 1/2 cup pineapple juice in reserve.
4. Mix the pulped pineapple, Splenda®, and Procel® in a large mixing tub, so you see no blobs.
5. Fold in a whipped cover, then put it aside. Boil the ½ cup pineapple juice in a shallow saucepan.
6. Connect 1 package of Knox® gelatin that is not flavored. Remove from heat and blend until dissolved. On graham crackers, add the mixture equally.
7. Place plastic wrap over the graham crackers from the edges of the pan.
8. Cover with foil made of aluminum and seal tight. Freeze overnight or for a period of 6 hours. "Cut into fifteen 2–1/2" by 2–1/2" bits until freezing and serve.

49. Watermelon Ice Cream

(Ready in about 3 hours | Serving 4 | Difficulty: Medium)

Per serving: Kcal 99, Fat: 1 g, Net Carbs: 20 g, Protein: 1 g

Ingredients:

- 3 cups cubed watermelon
- 2 medium frozen bananas
- 1 pinch sea salt
- ¼ tsp. vanilla extract
- 2/3 cup coconut milk
- 1 tbsp. honey

Instructions:

1. In a mixer, mix both ingredients and move to vacant ice cube containers.
2. Place them to freeze for 3 hrs or until they are frozen.
3. Carry the watermelon back to the processor.
4. Mix until it achieves a smooth texture.
5. Put the blend in a jar and bring it back to the freezer to stiff for approximately 25 mins or until the texture is needed.
6. Present like ice-cream with toppings needed.

50. Late Summer Blackberry Tart

(Ready in about 1 hour 25 minutes | Serving 6 | Difficulty: Medium)

Per serving: Kcal 236, Fat: 14 g, Net Carbs: 22 g, Protein: 3 g

Ingredients:

- 2/3 cup sliced plum

- 1 cup flour, unbleached

- 1 pinch sea salt

- 2 tbsp. regular sugar

- 1 egg

- 7 tbsp. cold butter

- 3 tbsp. cold water

- 2/3 cup blackberries

Instructions:

1. Preheat oven at 375°F.
2. Mix 1 tbsp. of sugar in a dish with blackberries and plum slices. Just set aside.
3. To yet another mixing dish, apply the remaining flour, salt, and sugar. Whisk in order to blend.
4. Using the fingers to split the butter till the combination is grainy like little peas.
5. Only before the mixture falls together, apply ice water, 1 tbsp. at one time. You don't want messy wet dough; just use enough to keep the dough intact.
6. For 20 minutes, and let dough settle.
7. On parchment paper placed over a flipside baking dish, spread the dough out. A rustic, rough edge would be the result.

8. In the middle, organize the fruit appealingly.
9. Bring the sides together, securing them by pressing the dough.
10. With 1 tbsp. of water, beat the egg.
11. Brush the egg wash on the tart dough. Sprinkle if needed with extra raw sugar.
12. Bake until thoroughly browned and crispy, around 30–35 minutes.
13. Serve it warm.

Conclusion

The main approach of this diet is to provide recipes that are not only easy to prepare but also a source for those that need extra care of their kidney functions. When you change to beneficial eating habits, you can experience how your renal activities ameliorate, and besides, your whole body gets better.

CPSIA information can be obtained
at www.ICGtesting.com
Printed in the USA
BVHW060910250321
603396BV00008B/579